Dom's Guide
To
Submissive Training
Vol. 2

25 Things You Must Know About Your
New Sub Before Doing Anything Else.
A Must Read For Any Dom/Master In
A BDSM Relationship

Elizabeth Cramer
Copyright© 2013 by Elizabeth Cramer

Copyright© 2013 Elizabeth Cramer
All Rights Reserved.

Warning: The unauthorized reproduction or distribution of this copyrighted work is illegal. No part of this book may be scanned, uploaded or distributed via internet or other means, electronic or print without the author's permission. Criminal copyright infringement without monetary gain is investigated by the FBI and is punishable by up to 5 years in federal prison and a fine of $250,000. (http://www.fbi.gov/ipr/). Please purchase only authorized electronic or print editions and do not participate in or encourage the electronic piracy of copyrighted material.

Publisher: Living Plus Healthy Publishing

ISBN-13: 978-1494390785

ISBN-10: 1494390787

Disclaimer

The Publisher has strived to be as accurate and complete as possible in the creation of this book. While all attempts have been made to verify information provided in this publication, the Publisher assumes no responsibility for errors, omissions, or contrary interpretation of the subject matter herein. Any perceived slights of specific persons, peoples, or organizations are unintentional.

This book is not intended for use as a source of legal, business, accounting or financial advice. All readers are advised to seek services of competent professionals in the legal, business, accounting, and finance fields.

The information in this book is not intended or implied to be a substitute for professional medical advice, diagnosis or treatment. All content contained in this book is for general information purposes only. Always consult your healthcare provider before carrying on any health program.

Table of Contents

Introduction 3

Level 1: Question 1 - 6 7

Level 2: Question 7 - 10 23

Level 3: Question 11 - 15 35

Level 4: Questions 16 - 20 49

Level 5: Questions 21 - 25 63

Conclusion 75

Introduction

There are two foundational pillars of a BDSM relationship between a Dom and a sub: **consent** and **trust**. Everything else in the relationship – the fun, the love, the discipline, the eroticism, the tears and the journey – are all built on those standards.

Both consent and trust require honest communication in order to thrive. The vast majority of that communication begins long before the training begins. Too often couples meet one another online or at a munch and jump straight into "What do you like?" or "Would you like to be my sub?" without asking crucial beginning questions. Those are fine if you are just doing some online play or a one night party spanking. But, when you are tired of that and are ready to create a long-term relationship with a devoted submissive, you need to ask questions that are deeper, more practical and helpful.

Many diverse traditions believe that questions have a high value in society and culture. Only when we ask do we cross the threshold of the door to wisdom. Ancient scholars maintain that students should be judged by their questions, not by their answers. A seeking, creative mind allows a Dom to give his sub the full attention, desire and best practices available in her training and life.

In a relationship built on power exchange, the act of asking questions is a gift the Dom gives his sub. It allows her to communicate freely and provides a mechanism for her to reveal her true self – even if she doesn't have the words to do so. There are a million things subs want their Doms to know. These questions will help your sub tell you.

The best way to ask someone a question is not to interview them, but ask questions at the appropriate time as part of a larger conversation (or email, in the case of online domination). Don't sit down with a list and a clipboard and grill your sub. Not only is that not sexy, but it would increase the pressure on her to perform (like someone would at an interview). The more she gets into performance mode, the less honesty will occur.

Some of these questions are very practical and do need to be asked right up front. Others are more subtle and open ended. They are specifically designed to get the sub to tell you her story or clue you into her depth of need and response. Ask the more subtle questions during casual talks as the topic arises. Listen to her answers and develop conversations around them.

Starting a relationship with the statement, "I'm the Master. Forget everything and just listen to me" is a sure fire way to create a momentarily exciting but frustrating short-term relationship headed for drama, disaster and end.

All women are different and come with many layers of history. Taking the time to gently unfold her secrets and truths will benefit your relationship greatly because you will have built up a strong foundation of trust that will endure. Show your sub you are a worthy Master not by what you tell her, but by what you ask her.

Note: If you are new to submissive training, be sure to read Volume 1 of this series: **"Dom's Guide To Submissive Training: Step-by-step Blueprint On How To Train Your New Sub. A Must Read For Any Dom/Master**

In A BDSM Relationship" available at all major book retailers.

Level 1: Question 1 - 6

1. What year were you born?

This is definitely the most important question for a practical reason, but it also offers the communication a chance to get off on the right foot. In all exchanges, especially online communication, you want to be sure the sub is actually a person over the age of 18 so you will not be in violation of international and national laws regarding child solicitation.

Talking about sexual things with an underage person is unwise for many reasons. First, she is a child and it is inappropriate to be sexual with a child. Second, you will be breaking the law and subject to serious penalties, including jail time and placement on the sex offender registry. Finally, it is possible you could be communicating with an investigator who is looking for child predators. If you do not make an active attempt to determine the age of the woman you are talking with, the case can be made that you were willing to be sexual with a child.

Do not ask, "How old are you?" Ask what year the sub was born. If you are instant messaging or in a chat room you should expect an instant answer. If you ask a sub their age, it is easy for them to lie and say quickly, "19." However, if you ask that person what year she was born and it takes a few minutes, then you know she went looking for a calculator or had to think about it. You shouldn't need to think about what year you were born. It should be an instant answer. That would be the first clue someone is lying about their age.

If someone sends you a private message on Tumblr, Fetlife, or Alt.com you won't have the advantage of watching how much time goes into the answer, but you can at least have an electronic record that you asked for the age of the sub.

If, for any reason, the sub changes her age while you are communicating with her and the new age falls under 18, even by a day, you need to discontinue the conversation no matter how enticing or desirable she seems.

For example: an online sub has told you she is 19, but a few messages later says, "Please don't be mad. I'm really 17 but I have a birthday next month so when we meet I will be legal." You should tell her immediately that you do not communicate with anyone under 18 and you will talk to her in a month when you see some kind of proof (driver's license, etc.) of her real age. A common rouse investigators use is to entice the suspect into a conversation then reduce the age to under legal standing.

Lying about age doesn't just happen with young folks who want to get in the game. Older women lie too, usually to make themselves appear younger, thinking it will make them more appealing.

While there is nothing illegal about saying you're 45 when you're really 52, it is better to start off every relationship with honesty. If she doesn't tell you the truth about her age, it will be harder for her to open up about other things as well.

Make sure your sub knows age is not an issue once legality is established and encourage her to start off with the truth.

2. What is your relationship status?

As much as possible, avoid asking simple "yes or no" or questions. If you ask your sub, "Are you married?" all she needs to tell you is "yes" or "no." For men who don't want to be involved with a married woman, the "yes" is all they need to hear. However, there is a lot more to her story than a simple answer, and if you intend to have a long-term Dom/sub relationship with her you need to hear it.

There are also too many variations to the word "married" that need to be fleshed out in your conversation. Let's say you ask your sub are you married, and she answers, "No." You think, "Great! She's mine!" But any one of the following could be true:

1. She is married but they haven't had sex with each other in years so she doesn't consider herself married. She's looking for something on the side to replace the sexuality she's missing. She doesn't intend to leave her husband and will need to meet at your place.

2. She is divorced from her husband but they are still living in the same house and enjoying a "friends with benefits" relationship

for the sake of the kids. So, she is free to offer her submission to someone, but she has someone else to go home to each night and the public still thinks they are a married couple.

3. She is getting ready to leave her possessive or abusive husband so she considers herself not married because she is already thinking of herself in the future. So, when you begin with the relationship you spend a lot of time dealing with an angry soon-to-be-ex-husband who follows you, causes trouble, or drags all of their marital drama into your life.

4. She lives with a boyfriend but they are not married. She is seeking a spanking or side-venture and hiding the fact from her boyfriend.

5. Her husband has died and she is coming to you out of grief. That may not mean you shouldn't want to have a relationship, but you should be aware if her submission is a grief decision.

Asking for her relationship status gives her a chance to explain things so you get a clear

11

picture of the situation and can make plans accordingly.

3. What is your living situation?

Just because a submissive woman doesn't have a husband does not mean she is living alone or has an unencumbered life. Try to get a full picture of what her living environment is like to make the decision about the type of submission you want to accept from her.

A single woman may have children who live with her. If that is the case, you need to factor in the ability to get private time without the children for your play plans. A woman with two teenagers in the house isn't going to be able to engage in 24/7 slavery. If she doesn't have custody of her children, she may get them every other weekend, or for the two weeks of Christmas. It's important to know what her life and time constraints are.

No woman lives in a vacuum. Some subs may have elderly parents who live with them or spend a large amount of time in their house. Others may have sisters getting divorced who are living there for a few months or roommates to help meet expenses.

Knowing exactly who is in the house will help you make better decisions in respect to your privacy and plans. You wouldn't want to send a bouquet of roses with a riding crop in it to her house if your sub's mom is going to answer the door. The less awkward your relationship is in public the smoother it will be in the bedroom.

Beyond living quarters, it is always good to know what other commitments your sub may have. Does she have elderly parents in a nursing home who require time and care? Is she a volunteer for the local animal shelter and spends a gallon of time walking dogs? Is she on a foster care list which means at any time a child may be assigned to come live with her that would change the whole dynamic of your relationship?

None of these things would prevent her from being a good submissive partner. However, it is hard for you to be a confident and competent Dom if you don't know what her life is like.

4. Can you describe what you look like?

If you are meeting online, never ask this question in the first thirty minutes. It is a sure way to get someone to click "End" or worse "Ban." From the sub perspective, if you ask that question too soon, it feels like she is automatically being judged or you only want her if she is a certain body type.

All women struggle with body image issues. If you approach a sub online and immediately start asking for pics she is going to think you are only out for a spanking model and wouldn't be interested in her. If she thinks that, she will cut you off before you get a chance to explain anything or before she gets a chance to know you.

Many Doms have a "type" that they are more attracted toward. Some men like BBW's and others prefer height/weight proportionate. There are shorter men who don't like to dominate very tall women and there are tall men who desire shorter women.

It is not wrong for you to seek out the type of woman that arouses you. It would be unhelpful if you picked a woman who did not stimulate you visually and gain your interest. The key is knowing how to ask that question.

Don't settle for just asking for a picture. Ask her first to describe herself. Ask what color her hair is or if she wears glasses. If she mentions that she drives a small car, ask her if she is tall. Lean the conversation toward her appearance.

The benefit to asking her to describe herself means you also get an idea of what part of her body she likes or dislikes. If she says, "I have really big boobs and I hate them." You can help her esteem by saying, "That's a shame. I bet they are wonderful." This also tells you that when you meet you should pay attention to other parts of her body first since she is uncomfortable with her breasts.

Eventually, you will need to meet her or see a picture. If this is going to be a long distance relationship for a while, do not settle for just whatever picture she sends you. Anyone can go on the internet and nab someone's vacation photos or Facebook album and send it. The same goes for nude pictures. The internet has no shortage of nude women for someone to use as a replacement for themselves.

The best thing to do is ask her to take a picture with a specific set of parameters. Ask for a picture of your sub in a red shirt wearing black pants and holding the day's newspaper.

Having your sub hold the newspaper is a great way to verify it is a recent picture by the date on the front page. This not only gives the sub an order to follow, but will help you feel confident you know with whom you are communicating.

If she claims not to have a camera or no one to take a picture of her (she can always take a selfie), or comes up with a list of excuses it is highly possible you are being catfished.

Most importantly, no matter what her answers are to the question, make sure when she describes herself or sends a picture that you are complimentary and sincerely appreciative of her as a sub. Praise her willingness to be vulnerable in sharing the details of her appearance. In return, make sure to send her a new and accurate picture of yourself as well.

5. Where have you lived?

Asking someone where she currently lives is a convenient way to discover her location. However, asking about a history of all the places she has lived will tell you much more about her experiences, environments and life story.

Knowing where someone lives is helpful in making plans for sessions or determining whether you will ever be able to meet in person. It's also great to know so you can accommodate any time differences (you don't want to call her at noon and discover it's 3 AM where she lives), and be aware of any laws or concerns if she lives in a different country than you.

Knowing how many places she has lived will live a wealth of information about her abilities, attitudes and experiences. If your sub was born and raised in one town, went to college there and lives there still, you can be reasonably sure she is not going to move to your location in a matter of months to be your 24/7 servant. You will also realize that she has deeply entrenched roots in her area which means she is less likely to be "out" about her fetish lifestyle and more concerned about privacy and safety.

No one wants to be asked to walk through the grocery store in short shorts showing a spanked bottom when she's worried about seeing her third grade teacher who goes to the same church as her aunt Mary.

People who stay in one place are also less experienced in other cuisines, music, images or culture from other places. In terms of discipline, someone from the Midwest of the United States who has never moved won't understand things like the British Disciplinary system (6 of the best) or eastern rituals.

By contrast, a submissive who has moved around a lot in her life is much more willing to consider relocation and tends to seek out new experiences more readily. She may have experienced a variety of foods, cultures, discipline styles or sexual attitudes.

People who have re-located a lot, particularly as children, often have the ability to make "fast friends" but don't connect deeply with anyone because they fear the person will leave or be "ripped away" from their life.

The sub's proximity to family and life-long friends is also good information to have so you know who and where her support system can be found in case she needs extra help or care.

6. What do you do?

Leave this question as broad as possible and encourage her to give you several answers in different areas of her life. In the United States people tend be very work oriented and identify themselves by their job. Submissives often offer their service to get away from their job and work persona and don't want to be identified by their profession.

A woman who is a business executive frequently offers her service as a submissive in order to balance out the power in her professional life with the powerlessness of her sexual life. So, she doesn't want to talk about her work or bring it into her submission. By asking "what do you do?" you give her the choice to limit or explore her other power position.

It is also helpful to know more about your submissive than what her favorite paddle is and how she makes money. Ask about things such as hobbies, interests and passions she may have. You can learn a lot about a sub by examining the types of things she likes to do with her spare time.

If she goes out to clubs, volunteers at community centers and spends weekends at the beach with a group of friends, you can see she is a very social person. Social subs do not do well locked into a training routine with a Master that doesn't involve time out and about around people. You would want to make sure all of your plans include some vanilla times with friends or allow her to experience service with a group of people (a munch, convention or play party) so her need to be social can be fulfilled.

If your submissive likes to do things like read, stay at home and watch TV, or put together puzzles, you will want to make a lot of your experiences private to help her feel more comfortable. Introverted subs don't dislike other people. Being around other people exhausts them. So, you may want to make sure a munch or play party is followed by a lot of down time or a chance for her to renew her energy.

An introverted sub will want to have focused experiences that are limited to the two of you. She may be challenged to serve other people while you watch, however, she will not be as comfortable or fulfilled as when she is alone with you.

Interests also tell you a great deal about things you can employ in your training and dominance. If your sub likes music, you can use some background music to inspire her giving or service. If she enjoys building and designing things, enlist her to help draw up plans for a new spanking bench or allow her to help you in the garage when you build new implements or furniture to use in her submission. There is nothing more delicious than being spanked with a paddle you selected the wood for or painted.

The more you understand about what your sub does when she is not focused on you – the better a match you will make in the long run.

Level 2: Question 7 - 10

7. Do you have any health concerns I should know?

The human body is an amazing thing. It is able to give and receive pleasure, process information at lightning speed, and move in wonderful ways. However, everyone's body is different and some folks have health issues you should know about.

Having a health concern, either physical or emotional, does not keep a woman from being a great submissive or mean there are things she can't do. Knowing her health history can help you make sure the play and training you design fits in with her best abilities and doesn't accidentally lead to harm or distraction.

Just because you don't see anything wrong doesn't mean there aren't things you need to know. Does she have problems with her joints or knees that might make you want to limit the time she spends kneeling? Are there back issues that require her to have lumbar support for an OTK spanking? Arthritis, muscular tension or previously wounded areas should all be things you are aware of and have factored into your plans.

Beyond physical disability, make sure to gather information on things such as allergies, blood sugar concerns (you don't want to have her tied up in a 3 hour rope session then discover her blood sugar is dropping and she needs to eat immediately), any history of blood pressure problems (bondage cuts off circulation and extended arousal such as orgasm denial increases heart rate), or breathing concerns.

Any submissive who has been treated in the past or is currently being treated for a diagnosed mental illness or cognitive disorder should also give you that information. The effects of a new relationship of submission and the intensity of training are sometimes overwhelming. If your submissive has experienced depression or is vulnerable to an affective disorder, knowing that fact can enable you to watch for signs and get her help as soon as possible.

If you are frustrated your submissive can't focus on one thing very long, or has trouble serving in silence, awareness she has ADHD will help you be more patient and construct a more helpful environment for you both.

Mental illness or cognitive disorders are not something your sub should feel ashamed of or afraid to disclose. The latest health statistics in the United States show 15% of adults have been treated or are currently in treatment for mental illness.

The beauty of being a submissive is learning to live without shame under the protection of your Master. Teaching your sub to openly discuss her concerns empowers her to trust and lean on you as a Dom worth serving.

8. When was your last test for sexually transmitted infections?

This isn't the sexiest question on the list, yet it is one of the most important. She may list herself as D & D (Drug and Disease Free) on her profile but if she hasn't been tested or she has had several sexual partners since her last test there is the potential for her to have a sexually transmitted infection (STI).

With the exception of HIV (which has no symptoms), men typically shows signs of STI very early in the disease process. Women, on the other hand, have the potential to be asymptomatic. That means they don't get sores, burning or any indication they have an STI but they still have the infection and are able to transmit it to you through any kind of sexual contact.

Don't just ask, "Have you been tested?" The easy "yes" doesn't give you any indication of when she was tested. Beware of the answer, "No, but I've only been with my husband." Since you have no way of knowing who else her husband may have been with, there is a risk of infection.

The best idea with a new submissive is to for both of you get tested at the same time. Most cities have free testing for STI's by the health department. Of primary importance is to be tested for HIV. The period of clinical latency for HIV is up to 10 years (you can have it for up to 10 years before you have symptoms).

If you and your partner are not tested, there will be no way of knowing whether or not you have the infection. With medication, HIV is a treatable illness. Without medication, HIV will become AIDS, with is fatal without care.

The other disease you want to ask specifically about and be tested for is Herpes. Herpes is not a fatal disease; however it cannot be cured with medication – only treated. The virus is only visible during an outbreak when genital or oral sores can be seen. The disease can be transmitted even when your partner is not having an outbreak. Always use a condom or barrier protection method if your partner has Herpes. If your partner is not currently experiencing an outbreak they can easily lie to you about their disease status. Getting tested for herpes is the best choice.

All other STI's can be cured with medication. If you have an STI and do not seek treatment you could be at risk for long-term effects that lead to infection, organ degeneration or death.

Seek treatment at the first sign of any STI and notify any sexual partners you have had about the possibility they may have been exposed to an infection. In the United States the local health department will notify people for you if that is something you don't want to do.

Clearly, it is always better to be tested for a disease and prevent it than need to be treated after the fact. Asking this question shows your sub that you care about your health, which makes her more likely to trust you will care about hers as well.

9. What are your limits?

Beware of any woman who comes to you and says, "I have no limits." She is either in fantasy land or is a poser. Every person has limits. A woman who is willing to say she would do anything her Master commanded without question is a woman who is likely to end up in prison or the grave. This question should be asked in such a way as to encourage your sub to admit she does have limits and facilitate an honest discussion about what they are.

Subs are often afraid to talk about their limits early in the relationship because they fear if they have too many limits a Dom might not choose them. There is also the fear that the Dom might see the limits as a challenge and try to make the sub do things she never wanted to do without proper consent and build up. When asking this question it is best to explain to your sub that there are two kinds of limits: hard limits and soft limits.

Hard limits are things that the submissive will not do and no amount of negotiation is going to change her mind. These are the things she will never consent to or consider. As her Master, you should also have a list of hard limits. Things that are morally wrong by all cultural standards and prohibited by law usually make up the bulk of hard limits.

Sex with children, sex with animals, rape or acts that do not involve consent, crimes, or entertainment that utilizes actual rape or death to achieve sexual arousal are all things that should be hard limits for you both. Other hard limits might include such things as permanent bodily damage or marking (tattoos, branding, scarification) or cause damage to your sub's reputation or employment (public humiliation, things that might lead to arrest).

Soft limits are things the submissive has chosen not to do because of lack of experience, fear or opportunity. A woman who has never had anal sex may list that as a limit. Over time, with trust and progress, she may change her mind about the practice. Submissives frequently find the idea of "water sports" to be a repulsive act they would never attempt. However, in the subspace mindset where they are enjoying being a pleasing servant they may decide that they want to please their Master by accepting his urine.

A soft limit is still a limit and should not be attempted until your sub has given consent to the act. All subs come with a little "wiggle room" in their list of things they will and will not do. Helping to clarify which acts may someday be added to your roster with experience, time and trust will give you a good list of challenges to work on.

10. What are religious/spiritual ideas and traditions?

All people are raised with some kind of religion or spiritual tradition. Even people raised with no religion or in atheist households are brought up in a system of thought about what might or might not be the order and spirit of the universe. Religion is a central part of every person's core being and will have a lot to do with how that person thinks, acts and reacts.

Fortunately, most people branch beyond the religion they are raised in to accommodate new thoughts and ideas as they grow older. Because BDSM is such a deep experience, many women will have added their philosophy and feelings of submission to their spiritual ideology. For some women, being a slave or a submissive is a spiritual truth they are following. For others, it is just a bedroom exercise.

Understanding your sub's spirituality will give you an excellent roadmap into what makes her tick. If she was raised in a conservative religious environment where God is a judgmental deity who is always on the lookout for what you are doing wrong, she is more likely to be discouraged by mistakes and constant discipline. You will need to take care during training to ensure she understands corrections and discipline is all part of obedience training and that you love and forgive her even when something goes wrong.

Sometimes women from conservative backgrounds have been taught that things like oral sex, anal sex, or polyamory are sinful and wrong. Working with her to broaden her view of spirituality will help those types of service move from the soft limit list to a possibility.

If your submissive has been raised in a very liberal environment where God isn't an issue or doesn't care what she does, she will be more likely to crave a strict and unrelenting Master. Many women raised without discipline and rules often crave a man who is willing to "lay down the law" and enforce a rigid code or structure for her to live within. She will look to you to provide those walls and building blocks and more readily accept rituals and punishments. Often subs who crave structure see discipline and guidance as evidence of love.

No matter what your sub believes about spirituality, it is better for you to work within her frame of reference rather than try to change her religious beliefs. Submissives who were raised conservative but have chosen to become atheists are not likely to re-embrace a God concept. Likewise, women who have chosen in their adulthood to follow a strict religious code will not abandon its practices because her Master wants something different.

You should develop a training and Dom/sub philosophy that encompasses both of your beliefs to move forward in positive directions.

Level 3: Question 11 - 15

11. When was your Aha! Moment?

One of the best parts of meeting a new sub is learning her story. There are only so many definitions of what it means to be a Dom or a sub, but the stories of how we end up at the truth of our nature are endless. Every life journey that brings a sub voluntarily to her knees is a collection of important firsts and moments that all lead her to kneeling in front of you. The Aha! Moment is that time when a submissive woman realizes that serving and being dominated is a part of her sexual identity.

For some women the Aha! Moment comes when they are very young, before they are old enough to engage in sex or submission. They may read about a character in a book who is dominant or discover her favorite Disney characters are the princesses who give loving devotion to their prince or the princes who take charge of the situation. Many women with a spanking fetish will talk about how they were captivated by the threat of a spanking they saw as a teen on a TV show, or how they were intrigued when someone was punished in a movie.

If you find a submissive whose story indicates she has always had these ideas, you have encountered a "natural submissive." Women who fit this category often think their submission is inborn and part of their fate. They think serving a man is at the very core of their being. When you are dominating them you need to be aware that nothing is a game to them. They take everything very personally. You aren't just dealing with "what they do"; you are dealing with "who they are."

For other women, awareness of their inclination to the bottom half of the equation comes later in life. They may meet a boyfriend in college or graduate school who has a spanking fetish and discover they find the sensations pleasurable. Some people don't begin until mid-life when a need for change or a new lover or an experience leads them to discover their submission.

Many times women will start to be interested in submission, read books, play online and learn all about the community for years before actually seeking a Master or getting spanked for the first time. Women who discover their submission later in life are more able to separate their identity from their pleasures. They tend to practice their submission in the bedroom only, or on a session basis and are much less likely to be "lifestylers."

Asking about a sub's Aha! Moment shows her you are interested in much more than using her body; you care about her identity and understandings as well. It gives you a solid foundation to build upon. Make sure to tell her about the moment you knew you had a dominant nature or enjoyed being a Master. Sharing who you were at the beginning of your journey will help your individual roads come together to form one path.

12. At what age did you get your first non-parental spanking?

Spanking isn't the only element in a Dom/sub relationship and most would argue it isn't the most important element, but it ranks near the top as one of the primary things that makes BDSM distinct. For a submissive, particularly one who has a lot of power in her outer world (work, home, family), spanking is the thing that allows her to strip (literally) away all of the responsibility and position she is clothed in and frees her to be vulnerable to another.

There is always a humiliating aspect to spanking an adult woman. She is being reduced from an empowered woman to being treated like a child, having her bottom bared and punished. An adult getting a bare bottom spanking or standing on display showing her red behind is a transformational experience. You should learn as much about your sub's first experience as possible.

The other reason to ask what age your sub was first spanked is to help you understand more of what her real time experiences have been. It is not uncommon for a Dom to meet a sub on a forum or in a chat room and ask how long she has been a sub. She will answer five years or more. If the Dom asks about her experience she might say she has served 3 Masters over the last 5 years and is now looking for a long-term Master. But, when you ask her what age her first actual non-parental spanking was she might just tell you she's never had one because all of her service has been online. Before you put a sub over your lap for a spanking you are going to want to know if it is her first.

If you meet a sub who has been serving in real time for a long time and has endured plenty of erotic and discipline spankings, it will still help you to know when she first started experiencing physical submission as opposed to fantasizing or serving online. Her early experiences in submission will frame much of her later experiences and may explain some of her likes, dislikes and attitudes about spanking.

Being involved with an online Master is a part of many women's story and is filled with heartfelt service and real feelings. But, it is not the same as the feeling she will get when your hand connects with her bottom for the first time.

13. What do you think a Dom/sub relationship involves?

Nothing creates more frustration than misunderstood roles, nothing creates more confusion than two people having a different definition of the same word, and nothing kills a relationship faster than unmet expectations.

Very early in your process you are going to need to understand what your sub thinks the dynamics and roles in your relationship are going to be. There may be a lot of books out there about BDSM but there is no authoritative definition of what the relationship is going to look like, function like or feel like. Every person has their own ideas.

Not only does each sub and Dom have unique expectations about what is going to happen in the relationship, but each also has their set of "right and wrong" they have learned through their experiences in submission. You may encounter a sub who had a Daddy Dom previously and thinks a Dom who doesn't do a lot of aftercare is being emotionally abusive. This will clash with your methods if you believe a sub should not receive aftercare when she gets a discipline spanking because it is supposed to hurt. Some subs think a Dom must always follow the "hurt but not harm" mantra, and others think a Dom is supposed to challenge you all the way to the edge of your ability.

Deep differences in philosophy can make training extremely difficult and create a chasm of communication in which the intentions of the Dom to structure the relationship are challenged or misunderstood.

If your sub feels a Dom is a protector and teacher she may be shocked if you offer her to another Dom, or expect her to know how to serve without a lot of instruction or help. If you approach a Dom/sub relationship with an emphasis on domestic service, high protocol and absolute obedience you are going to be very frustrated with a sub who likes to brat, play around and doesn't take her chores or demeanor very seriously.

One of the keys to this question is discovering how your sub feels about the idea of submission as a lifestyle. Subs who believe that the Dom/sub relationship is a lifestyle will expect to be in the role of sub all the time. They want a Master who is "always on" and providing structure, answers, and directions at all times. They will be more likely to give over total control and expect the Master to carry the weight of the relationship on his shoulders. Subs who are session subs don't expect the Master to rule all the time and aren't ready to live in a submissive role 24/7. If you approach a session sub with ideas about constant submission, one of you is going to be disappointed.

Take time to listen carefully to her answer to this question and make sure your ideas of what you want to be as a couple are compatible with what she is thinking. Often a Dom may agree to a sub's ideas of the relationship because he wants her to be his sub and thinks he can change his ideas to accommodate her needs. Within a few weeks, he is back to thinking his usual way and she is angry that he is "changing the game" now that time has passed.

If you don't have an initial compatible view of what a Dom/sub relationship is like, resolve to be supportive friends and align yourself with someone more similar.

14. What were some of your best experiences as a submissive?

Sometimes nothing can be more tedious than listening to a sub talk about what she has done with other Doms. It can bring up insecurities about how you are going to "measure up" or add pressure to an already delicate situation.

Don't worry. If she wanted to be with that other Dom, she would. She is talking to you because she is interested in giving her service and body to you. Learning what some of her best experiences have been in the past is worth enduring the tales because it gives you a chance to pick up on the things that are effective without her having to tell you.

For example: a sub tells her new Dom, "I like things that are very sweet and romantic." When the Dom brings her flowers she isn't going to get as much joy because she told him that's what she wants. It's like going to a store and picking out your own Christmas gift. However, if she tells you one of her best experiences was when her Dom went out of his way to go to her office and left a rose in her car for her to find after work, you will figure out she likes romantic gestures and be able to come up with some neat ways to shower her with romance.

Keep the question open to hearing about more than one experience. The more information she gives you the greater your ability to see different facets of her personality. If you hear the rose story you might be tempted to think she is all romance. But, if the next story she tells you is about her first experience with a single tail whip and how she loved the bruising it left on her the next day, you'll understand that while she might enjoy a touch of the soft stuff, she also enjoys a great deal of pain and lingering after effects. If the two stories are linked together and she got the rose the day after she endured her first single tail lashing, you'll be able to see she likes to be rewarded or appreciated for enduring pain and new experiences.

Sometimes the things people remember as a good experience will surprise you. You might have a sub you think you understand pretty well as a private sub who keeps her submission a secret, only to discover one of her best experiences was being spanked at a rest stop where another adult could see the event. She may be as surprised as you about how erotic that experience felt to her.

Discussing the good times will sometimes not only tell you about your sub, but also help her do some introspective thinking about her own desires.

15. What have been some of your worst submissive experiences?

It's no fun to listen to the good times your sub had with other Doms, but it's definitely not pleasant to hear the painful things she has been through at the hands of another. Just as learning her good experiences will help you understand your sub, learning about her bad and painful experiences will give you a wealth of knowledge to both instruct and heal her.

When a submissive woman puts her body and soul on the line with a Master she is taking a great risk. Unfortunately, not all men who call themselves "Master" are worthy of service and some are abusive. A submissive woman in a bad relationship can be physically harmed, emotionally damaged, or completely broken by an abusive Dom. If that has been the case, you need to know as much as you can about those experiences.

You don't want to do anything that might bring back the memory of those experiences or damage her trust any further in that area. If a Dom showed up at your sub's workplace and acted inappropriately, she may be frightened to tell you where she works, or fearful if you suggest you will pick her up for lunch. It takes time and a collection of new experiences to heal from a bad one. The more gently you go about that part of the process, the better.

Not all bad experiences come from abusive Doms. Sometimes subs just end up with a Dom who didn't have good communication skills or acted in a way that fit within the protocol of a Dom/sub relationship but didn't meet her needs or expectations.

For example, some submissive women don't cry tears when they are spanked. If a Dom is giving her corporal punishment and hasn't communicated with her enough to know she is not someone who is going to cry, he may actually take the spanking too far and end up harming her because he is waiting for her tears to fall. If there wasn't a safe word in place, that would lead to a terrible experience for the sub.

Training and a lot of upfront communication are necessary to make sure these kinds of events don't happen. By learning about the bad experiences your sub has endured you will be a Dom who is wiser and better equipped to train her into your service.

Level 4: Questions 16 - 20

16. What are your triggers (good and bad)?

Both good and bad experiences can create a memory "trigger." A trigger can be anything – sound, feeling, touch, taste, smell, or situation that brings up a memory of a former experience. Once the memory returns the sub will relive that memory and will create a lens through which she sees or understands the current event.

For example, if anal sex was a limit your sub had but her Dom forced her into it without her consent, she may feel your attempts to approach the subject are the same as the anal rape she endured and shut down completely. Even though you are not harming her, she will see your efforts through the lens of her past pain.

Triggers can often be brought on by certain toys or similar situations. Sometimes a sub won't even realize something is a trigger until she encounters the situation a second time. If your sub had a Dom who used a lexan paddle on her so hard it surpassed her pain limit and damaged her, she might agree to let you use a lexan paddle, but then react in an unexpected way because she is living with the former memory.

If she starts to fight you, pull away or use her safe word at an unexpected time, chances are the trigger memory is interfering with her current session. Fortunately, few subs experience so many bad events that they have a long list of triggers. Most will have left their abusive Dom quickly and resolved some of their pain or issues before trying again. Still, painful memories can be devastating if they are not healed or acknowledged.

Not all memory triggers are bad or come from bad events. All humans have things that bring good feelings and good memories to them as well. Good triggers are fantastic to know because you can utilize those feelings to reward and nurture your sub.

Don't just ask about good feelings from fetish encounters. Ask about all the things that bring her fond memories or make her feel good. If the smell of bread baking in the oven is something that calms your sub or makes her happy, you can reward her by baking some bread before she arrives.

Subs who are forty years old and older are more likely to have been raised with physical discipline and told that they were being spanked because a parent loved them. If your sub's father used a wooden paddle on her as a child, and connected the fact he spanked her with love, she may want you to use a wooden paddle for maintenance spankings to show your love to her as well.

The final thing to remember about triggers is that when you are with your submissive everything you do has the power to make triggers as well. Punishment or reward, sex or stimulation, high protocol or casual – you are making memories with your submissive every day and some of those are going to last. Tell her it is your goal to leave good memory triggers for her and heal the bad ones.

17. On a scale of 1 to10, how much pain is pleasant, arousing, and too much.

Every person has a different idea of what constitutes pain. In medicine they judge pain in patients by having people tell them what their pain feels like on a scale of 1 to 10. Since some people find a paper cut to be a 1 and others might find it a 5 – the pain scale lets medical professionals know how much pain the patient feels without having to worry about how to define their ability to feel pain.

Much in the same way, every sub you encounter will have a different response to physical pain and a different reaction to the levels of pain they experience. Subs can range anywhere from a tenderfoot who can barely take the sting of a hand spanking to a pain pig who experiences arousal at skin-ripping whip lashes. Most subs will be somewhere in the middle of that scale.

By asking your sub to rate her feelings about pain and her reaction to each level of pain you will be much better equipped to design experiences and punishments that are effective. You always want to push and challenge your sub's pain limits, but you want to do it in small steps so you don't overwhelm her and cause her to pull away. Even a disciplinary spanking must have the right amount of pain to be instructive but not over-the-top.

Not all submissive women find spanking pleasurable, although the vast majority are attracted to physical pain at some level. It's important to discover the spectrum of pain to which your sub assigns her feelings and reactions.

Ask her, using the 1 to 10 scale how much pain she finds pleasant and get an example of what might cause that level. Most submissives find pain levels 1 and 2 to be pleasant – for many that means a pinkish to red bottom from a hand/paddle spanking, light bondage in comfortable positions, or oral or vaginal sex when she is aroused and well lubricated.

After you discuss pleasure, ask what level of pain leads to her sexual arousal. Arousal is usually one or two steps after her pleasure level. For many subs that will be a 4 or 5 – a deep red or welted bottom with a leather paddle, hairbrush or tawse, bondage that is restricting but a comfortable position (breast bondage, hands or legs tied down), or anal, vaginal or rough oral sex (face fucking) when she is aroused and lubricated.

Finally ask her where on the scale the pain becomes intolerable. What level of pain makes her experience go from good to bad or creates a sense of panic or need for her to use her safe word and end the session? For many subs the 8 to 10 pain range includes whippings or beatings that cause bleeding, welting or skin tears – canes, single tail whips, crops, floggers, bondage in unnatural or uncomfortable positions for a long period of time, or anal or vaginal sex without proper lubrication or arousal.

18. What do you like best – anticipation, action or afterglow?

Everyone has a favorite part of submission or session experience. Some women are all about the anticipation of the event. A sub who finds the most pleasure in imagining and thinking about what is going to happen will play scenarios over again and again in her mind. She imagines the humiliation of taking her clothing off, the lecture or instruction, the moment your hand touches her bottom, the first sting of pain, the taste, the sex, and the afterglow. Ruminating on all that is going to happen gives her sexual pleasure and fulfillment.

Subs who like the days and hours building up to a session need a lot of pre-attention. Send your sub emails each day reminding her that soon she will be OTK or telling her that you can't wait to accept her service. Tease and tantalize her a little bit. Make sure to meet most of her expectations (after all, she's been planning this for days) but also add in some surprises and twists so she isn't bored when she finally experiences the moment.

Submissive women who prefer the action of the actual event don't need as much care in the days preceding your session together, but they need your entire focus on them from the beginning to the end of the event. These women don't spend a lot of time in fantasy, and are much less likely to serve an online Dom for any length of time. What they want is the visceral feeling of being with you, having you strip and spank them (usually with a lot of ritual involved) and serving you with their body. They don't want to know any plans ahead of time and like to be caught up in the action.

For these women, make sure the phone is off and your distractions are at a minimum. Have everything you need for your session and know what your plan is going to be. Once you two start she isn't going to want you to stop until it's all over. Action oriented women are also far less in need of aftercare or interested in long afterglow. They are more likely to want to leave or change gears as soon as the session ends.

Afterglow is that period after your orgasm (and maybe hers) when you engage in aftercare – rubbing lotion on her wounds and sore buns – and give her a lot of hugging, attention, praise and nurture. Some people enjoy submission simply because of the afterglow period. They are more likely to want a Daddy

Dom, or someone to tell them how cherished they are and how well they did. They need a lot of positive affirmation.

When you realize the pain and service your sub has endured just to get to the part where you hug her and tell her how proud you are of her efforts, it shows you the afterglow period is truly important. Don't plan to end your session with only a few minutes left for goodbyes. Give yourself plenty of time for hugs and snuggles.

If your sub says she loves all three times equally – add an extra hour to your session plans and take a lot of vitamins – you're going to need them.

19. How much time do you spend naked?

Nudity is an incredibly important part of the submissive experience. Clothing has a lot of meaning and value in our society. The type of clothing you wear can tell people about your economic situation, status, interests identity and habits. Clothing can tease, deceive, shelter, protect and project personality. The act of taking off clothing is the act of stripping away all the layers of society and the social ideas that go with them.

Having a woman disrobe for your pleasure instantly changes her mindset as her power and position are taken off piece by piece. By the time you are ready to accept her submission a lot of the "world" will have been peeled away, leaving her vulnerable and ready for service.

Your sub should be open to you at all times and in every way. In training it is very practical to keep your sub naked so you don't have to deal with clothing every time you want to give her a few swats or at any time you want to use her body for your pleasure. Your sub should always be prepared, open, available and ready for you. So, it is very helpful if she is comfortable without her clothing; wearing nothing but her collar.

Knowing how much time your sub spends naked will also clue you in to how comfortable she is with her body and being vulnerable. A sub who walks around her house naked or is used to watching TV or doing chores naked won't be as agitated or self-conscious during her submission because she is used to seeing her own body. A sub who always wears clothing of some kind, including pajamas to sleep in, will be less natural in the beginning of her submission because she is hyperaware of her body and the fact that it is on display.

If your sub is nervous or cautious about nudity, you can use clothing as part of your reward system in the beginning. If you offer to allow her to wear a T-shirt or panties depending on how well she does a certain task, you can incorporate her need into your training regimen. When she tells you she wants to stay naked to please you, you will know your training is working well.

Most subs will say the more time they spend naked the more they enjoy the freedom of nudity and the less appealing it is to put on clothing. For those subs, the idea that they have to get dressed once the session is over, or that they have to put on clothes to go to work becomes the harder transition for them to make.

The more your sub is comfortable with her body, the more able she will be to devote it to you and to serving your needs. If you are working with an online sub in preparation for meeting, make sure you ask her to spend at least one hour a day doing something naked.

20. What do you think about when you masturbate?

In order for a woman to achieve orgasm her brain has to be fully involved in the process. That's why you want to spend so much time asking these questions. You want enough information to incorporate her brain and body into your structure.

When women masturbate fantasy is an important element in their ability to achieve release. So, all women fantasize or think about something that can bring them to the brink and push them over. Knowing what your sub runs through her mind before she reaches climax will show you how to please and arouse her with ease.

Subs are always thinking about giving the answer that will please the Master. It is likely when you ask this question she is going to say, "I think about you." Don't let her get by with such an obvious and easy answer. If she is thinking about you, or even if she is not, what is she thinking?

If she is running a fantasy through her head where you are on top of her, dominating her and calling her a slut or whore while you ram your cock into her body, then you know she is aroused by a sense of shame, humiliation and rough sex. If she is thinking about you kissing her and telling her how beautiful she is as she prepares for climax, then you know she needs a lot of romance and reinforcement to get turned on.

Our fantasies don't just tell us what we want in our secret hearts or private lives. They give us real time clues about the kinds of things that drive us forward and bring us to release. The more you learn about her thought process during sex and toward release the better you will be able to fulfill her fantasies and be the Master of her dreams.

Level 5: Questions 21 - 25

21. How do you communicate your needs?

Understanding your sub's communication patterns and habits absolutely needs to happen before you begin training. Once she submits herself to you and enters into her submission mode she will not be in a position to offer you a lot of answers or do a lot of constructive communicating. Her entire thought process will change to focus on pleasing you and saying whatever she thinks will make you happy. Plus, once she is over your lap with a gag in her mouth it isn't the best time to ask her deep or complex questions.

A submissive woman who is very articulate will be able to express her needs to you clearly through verbal communication. She can tell you if she feels challenged or if she thinks your sessions are setting her up to fail. She will be willing to tell you if her morning spankings are hard enough or whether she feels isolated in your service and needs to go out or be around more people.

For subs who are good at expressing their feelings and needs you need to set aside a time each day for a small listening period where she is free to talk about what's going on in her head.

Other women are not as good with verbal communication and will use other methods to try to let you know if something is right or wrong. Subs who use the silent treatment or pout in order to let a Dom know they aren't happy with something are very frustrating to work with. Often a Dom thinks the pouting is just an act or some bratting the sub is doing to get more attention and spanks her more, which creates a classic miscommunication.

Sometimes a sub will do extra chores or put extra energy into a project in order to show you her happiness and gratitude. If you don't notice that or realize it is how she communicates, you are likely to disappoint her.

In terms of limits and pain, there are submissive women who take their obedience training very stoically and don't tell you that you are actually causing them harm. They may endure the session, which you think went great, only to get home and write you an email telling you it was too hard and she no longer wants to serve you.

Sometimes a sub cries so often and loudly during a spanking that it is hard to tell if she is just into her session or trying to get you to stop. Having a discussion about whether your sub cries tears, kicks and screams or grows silent when the pain is reaching the limit is best done clearly and early in the process.

22. What kind of support system do you have?

It is very easy to think of submission in terms of you and your sub without anyone else being involved. However, your sub is going to need a much broader support network than you can offer by yourself.

Being a submissive partner is a tremendous stressor. Subs feel the internal stress of always wanting to please the Master and trying to find new ways to do things, as well as communicate her feelings. They also feel the external pressure of the rest of their obligations – jobs that need to be done, kids that need cared for, parents who ask a lot of questions, friends who want to be social – and they are trying to balance the needs of the others in their life with their desire to focus on you.

Submission, particularly in training, is emotionally grueling, physically painful, and exhausting. If she doesn't have some folks outside of your environment that she can blow off steam with, she is going to explode.

Allow your sub time each day to go on any of the online forums or websites that exist to support submissives. Don't be insecure about anything your sub might say or hear on these websites. These aren't groups for women plotting to overthrow Doms and ruin relationships. They are women who want to help each other be more pleasing and fulfilled by sharing experiences, ideas and encouragement. Your sub may have friends at work or be happy with her family, but she will need someone else to talk with who understands what it's like to be tied to a spanking bench and waiting for her punishment.

If you met your sub online and you are preparing for a meeting, make sure to ask her what safety protocol she intends to follow for meeting you. That way, even if you don't have good chemistry and it doesn't go anywhere, you will have taught her something valuable.

A sub should always have a safety person who knows where she is meeting you, what time, how long the meeting should last and how to reach you (an email address). She should set up a safety call when she arrives at the public place for your meeting and tell her safety person a time when the meeting is supposed to end so she can call again.

Most experienced subs will already have their support system in place. However, you can't access it or help her use it if you don't know what it is or who the principal players are in her support network.

23. What heals you?

This is both a physical and emotional question. All women have remedies, traditions or rituals they use to heal from the physical pain of BDSM and know secrets to help the bruising or welts clear up. A healing routine is like a beauty routine. If followed, everything will be fine. If ignored, someone is going to be upset!

Many women enjoy having their Dom rub lotion on their bottom after a hard spanking. However, if you use a strap, or a rope from bondage rubs off some skin, lotion would not be wise to use because it clogs pores and actually prevents healing.

Some women swear ice reduces welts quickly and use a 20 min. on, 20 min. off ice pack solution. Others use Icy Hot or Miracle Ice to stimulate circulation to help bruises disappear more quickly (without that greenish/brown period). Make sure you understand the best ways to help her recover from a rough session or hard beating.

Healing emotionally isn't as easy. Some subs come into your care already wounded. They may have suffered childhood abuse, grief, loss, rape or humiliation before you met them. You need to find out what they use to help them heal or manage to keep going.

If your sub uses guided imagery and meditation to help keep her bad memories away or clear the past stress from her life, you need to give her time to do that while in your service. If wine and chocolate help her overcome her sense of grief, stock up. When she sees you are interested in making sure he is as whole and healed as she can be, her heart will start healing from all that has come before.

Sometimes, even though it is not your intention, you may hurt your sub's feelings or create a physical or emotional wound yourself. Instead of just "trying what worked with someone else" make sure to ask her up front what kinds of things will help her understand your desire to make amends.

It can be hard for a Dom to apologize. However, for some subs, having a Dom who is willing to admit he made a mistake and wants to make amends is the best feeling in the world. Other subs may think that is a sign of weakness in a Dom and actually withdraw if you apologize. Ask your sub what is the best way for you both to create lines of communication that help you overcome mistakes (because you are human and they will happen) quickly and effectively.

Women don't just want men who are going to use them. They want a Dom who is going to own them, challenge them and heal them.

24. What do you get from submission?

In some ways a Dom/sub relationship seems to be a one way street. The Dom makes his desires and wishes known and the sub fulfills them. However, if that's all there was to this, more people would give it a try.

A Dom not only gets his way, he also has to take the responsibility for the relationship, maintain the parameters, structure the training and stay vigilant to the needs of the sub. What he gets, besides sexual pleasure, is a sense of fullness and happiness that he is providing the best direction for the relationship as possible.

A submissive does more than just bend, serve, strive and meet the needs of her Master. She needs to get something from the relationship as well. Ask your sub what she takes away from the arrangement.

Some women get a sense of honoring traditional roles that connects them to the past. Others feel the pride of meeting the challenges of submission and making it through. Still others feel they were born submissives and serving their Master well is a way to connect with her destiny. Many feel the release of stress, the freedom from being in charge, or just the fun of doing something different and taboo.

Whatever your sub gets from her service, make sure you understand what it is and set up scenarios where that feeling is assured.

Praise your sub and encourage her giving. When you go through a particularly rough session give her a lot of compliments when it is over about her ability to make it through and lift up the strength she has. Find ways to let your sub know she is pleasing to you and you are proud of her.

A Dom/sub relationship is never just about the needs of one person. Make sure she knows that, and make sure she knows that you know it too.

25. What do you expect in training?

Just as question number 1 was the first question you should ask every person, this question illustrates the transition from communication into your Dom/sub relationship. Asking your sub this question lets her know that things are moving forward. It also makes her very aware that training is not an option but a healthy and required part of a healthy relationship.

If your sub should tell you she has experience and she really doesn't need training, this is your chance to educate her in BDSM and let her know that you are not like any of the other Masters she has had in the past. She will need training to learn how best to submit to you, and it is something you will both enjoy and grow through.

Listening to her expectations gives you a really good idea of what she has actually experienced. If she claims to have been through training, but does not know what a submissive posture is, or isn't aware of how to serve a room, then you can see you need to work on her protocol.

Sadly, some subs come from experiences with substandard Doms whose training was limited to, "I'll give you a good hard spanking and put this collar on you and you're mine." If she expects to have a time of learning, limit pushing and challenge then you can tell she's had a training experience worthwhile.

Her answer can also clue you in on what kind of submissive experience she is expecting. If her vision of training includes a lot of sex and play but very little discipline or domestic service, she is really leaning more toward being a pleasure slave.

If she describes a high amount of caregiving, cooking, and tending to your needs and skips a lot of the sexual aspect – she is wanting more of a domestic slave/sub position. After you get a chance to hear her vision of what training will be like, tell her about your plans and structure and give her a roadmap of what her next few weeks will entail.

Conclusion

Questions don't simply lead us to answers. They lead us to new pathways, better journeys and an ability to see and understand each other in profoundly deep ways. The more you know about the woman who will be kneeling at your feet, the better Dom you will be for her. Always take the time to listen to your sub and if there is something you don't know or don't understand, ask her some questions. One of the best and most proud things a sub can say about her Dom is, "My Master is wise."

Other books by Elizabeth Cramer:

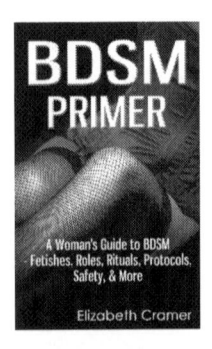

BDSM Primer - A Woman's Guide to BDSM - Fetishes, Roles, Rituals, Protocols, Safety, & More

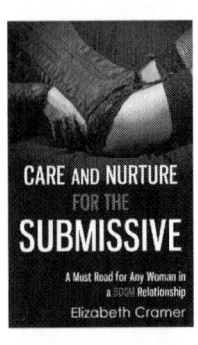

Care and Nurture for the Submissive - A Must Read for Any Woman in a BDSM Relationship

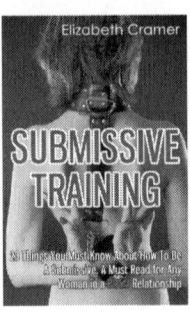

Submissive Training: 23 Things You Must Know About How To Be A Submissive. A Must Read For Any Woman In A BDSM Relationship

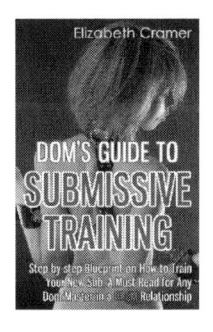

Dom's Guide To Submissive Training: Step-by-step Blueprint On How To Train Your New Sub. A Must Read For Any Dom/Master In A BDSM Relationship

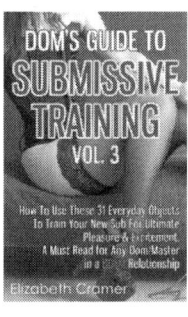

Dom's Guide To Submissive Training Vol. 3: How To Use These 31 Everyday Objects To Train Your New Sub For Ultimate Pleasure & Excitement. A Must Read For Any Dom/Master In A BDSM Relationship

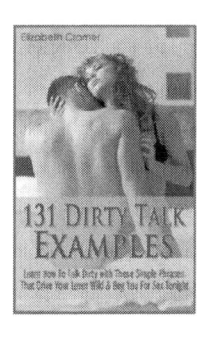

131 Dirty Talk Examples: Learn How To Talk Dirty with These Simple Phrases That Drive Your Lover Wild & Beg You For Sex Tonight

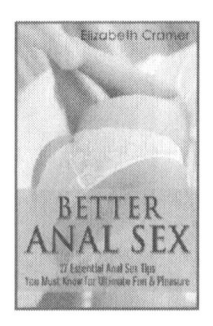

Better Anal Sex - 27 Essential Anal Sex Tips You Must Know for Ultimate Fun & Pleasure

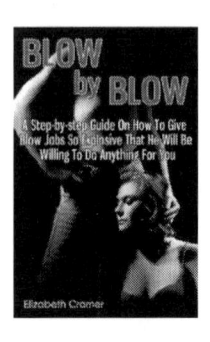

Blow By Blow - A Step-by-step Guide On How To Give Blow Jobs So Explosive That He Will Be Willing To Do Anything For You

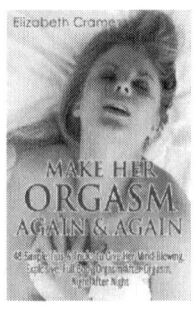

Make Her Orgasm Again and Again: 48 Simple Tips & Tricks to Give Her Mind-Blowing, Explosive, Full-Body Orgasm After Orgasm, Night After Night

Printed in Great Britain
by Amazon.co.uk, Ltd.,
Marston Gate.